BLADDER SURGERY RECOVERY DIET

Proven Surgical Techniques And Revitalizing Your Healing Journey For Optimizing Recovery And Bladder Health

DR LUCAS KAYCE

DISCLAIMER

This book about illness and nutrition is not meant to replace expert medical advice, diagnosis, or treatment; rather, it is meant purely for informational reasons. This book's content is founded on broad concepts and recommendations for managing diseases and nutrition.

Before adopting any major dietary or lifestyle changes, readers are recommended to speak with a qualified healthcare provider, such as a licensed physician or registered dietitian, especially if they have pre-existing medical concerns. Everybody has different health demands, so what works for one person might not work for another.

The use of the information provided in this book may have unfavorable repercussions or consequences, for which the author and publisher disclaim all liability. No disease is meant to be identified, treated, cured, or prevented by the information provided.

The book may include contain references to medical literature or research findings; however readers are urged to independently confirm this material and contact reliable sources.

It is important to remember that the fields of nutrition and medicine are always changing, and that new findings could have an impact on the advice offered in this book. As a result, readers are urged to keep up with the most recent advancements in healthcare and, when in doubt, seek professional counsel.

By reading this book, readers agree that they are in charge of their own health decisions and release the author and publisher from any liability arising from the use of the material in the book, whether direct or indirect.

TABLE OF CONTENTS

ABOUT THE BOOK

The "Bladder Surgery Recovery Diet" book is a thorough manual created to offer priceless insights into the complex connection between nutrition and the recuperation phase after bladder surgery. The introduction provides a basic overview of bladder surgery, explaining the many kinds and stressing the importance of a carefully planned recovery diet for the healing process.

An in-depth discussion of frequent problems and the critical role diet plays in promoting healing is provided, which also explores the subtleties of the bladder surgery recovery process. "Getting Ready for the Recovery Journey," provides helpful advice on eating before surgery, stressing the importance of being hydrated and being mentally ready.

"Post-Surgery Dietary Essentials, offers a comprehensive guide for the critical post-surgery phase. It describes basic nutritional rules, suggests foods that are soft and readily broken down, and emphasizes the significance of nutrient-dense choices. The next chapter, "The Bladder-Friendly Diet Plan," goes a step further, giving a thorough how-to for putting together a balanced meal plan, outlining what foods to include and what to avoid, and including sample meal plans for various phases of recovery.

Aspects of recovery are covered in detail, ranging from the management of typical post-surgery symptoms through diet to the need for exercise, nutritional supplements, and hydration. Every part has been carefully designed to provide useful guidance and recommendations that are supported by research.

The book also explores the emotional components of rehabilitation by highlighting the significance of having a strong support network, providing coping mechanisms, and examining the relationship between diet and mood. The book addresses long-term dietary issues, helping readers make the shift to a regular diet, upholding a healthy lifestyle, and putting strategies in place to track and stop recurrence.

The "Bladder Surgery Recovery Diet" is a comprehensive guide that addresses the various aspects of recovery and goes beyond a simple set of food recommendations. It combines practical counsel with a wealth of nutritional knowledge to empower readers as they embark on their path to maximum healing.

One of the most important medical interventions for treating urological disorders is bladder surgery, which entails performing surgical treatments on the urinary bladder. The diagnosis and treatment of conditions affecting the bladder, an essential organ that stores and eliminates urine from the body, are the focus of this subspecialty of surgery. When conservative measures are ineffective in treating symptoms or when anatomical anomalies necessitate surgical repair, bladder surgery becomes necessary.

BLADDER SURGERY TYPES

There are various kinds of bladder surgery, each intended to treat particular ailments and reduce associated symptoms. Transurethral resection of the bladder (TURBT) is a frequent treatment that involves removing malignant tumors from the bladder to treat the disease.

Bladder augmentation is a different operation that is frequently used to treat chronic bladder dysfunction or congenital anomalies. It entails enlarging the bladder to increase its capacity. Furthermore, when cancer or other serious illnesses require the removal of the bladder, urinary diversion procedures may be performed to redirect the urine's flow.

Other bladder surgeries include cystoscopy, a diagnostic surgery that uses a thin tube equipped with a camera to view the inside of the bladder, and cystectomy, which involves removing the bladder entirely. These surgeries, along with others, demonstrate the variety of therapies that can be used to treat various bladder-related problems.

DIET IS IMPORTANT FOR RECOVERY

It is impossible to exaggerate the importance of food in the healing process following bladder surgery. A diet that is high in nutrients and well-balanced is essential for bolstering the body's natural healing processes and enhancing general well-being.

Individuals undergoing bladder surgery are frequently recommended to adhere to particular dietary regimens to reduce risks, facilitate recuperation, and preserve optimal urinary health.

Drinking enough water after surgery is essential for preventing UTIs and facilitating the body's natural removal of toxins. Maintaining appropriate urine function and avoiding dehydration-related problems require consuming an adequate amount of water. A diet high in antioxidants, vitamins, and minerals also strengthens the immune system, promoting healing and lowering the chance of infection.

Dietary modifications may be required in cases where urinary diversion procedures have been performed to account for altered urine patterns. To prevent items that can irritate the urinary system or cause difficulties, patients may need to adjust their diet.

In addition, bowel function is influenced by food decisions, which is an important factor for people recuperating after bladder surgery. A diet rich in fiber promotes general digestive health and helps avoid constipation, a typical worry following surgery.

Both patients and caregivers must comprehend the many kinds of bladder surgery and the role that a well-balanced diet plays in the healing process. By going over these aspects in detail, people can better navigate the difficulties associated with bladder surgery by knowing what procedures are involved and what kind of aftercare is required for a speedy recovery.

CHAPTER ONE

COMPREHENDING THE RECOVERY PROCESS AFTER BLADDER SURGERY

AN OVERVIEW OF SURGERY ON THE BLADDER

Depending on the individual diagnosis, bladder surgery—a medical treatment frequently required by illnesses such as bladder cancer, urine incontinence, or bladder dysfunction—involves a variety of approaches. The main objective of bladder surgery is to treat and resolve problems that interfere with the bladder's natural function so that patients can take back control of their urinary system. Depending on the patient's needs, these surgical operations may use minimally invasive methods, open surgeries, or transurethral procedures.

Following bladder surgery, patients have a recovery period during which several parameters need to be carefully monitored. People frequently report feeling uncomfortable, in pain, or having trouble moving around in the early days after surgery.

Recovery times can change depending on the kind of surgery done, general health, and if there are any after-effects. Patients are usually urged to adhere strictly to post-operative instructions, which may include wound care, restrictions on physical activity, and using prescription drugs to control pain and avoid infection.

TYPICAL REHAB OBSTACLES

One of the main obstacles during the recuperation phase following bladder surgery is the possibility of complications like bleeding or infection. Early intervention depends on keeping an eye out for infection-related symptoms, such as fever, increased discomfort, or changes in urine color.

Furthermore, it's critical to strike a balance between rest and a gradual increase in physical activity to avoid difficulties and advance healing. During the healing process, patients are frequently urged to discuss any worries or strange symptoms with their healthcare practitioners openly and honestly.4

NUTRITION'S FUNCTION IN HEALING

To promote the healing process following bladder surgery, nutrition is essential. The body's capacity to heal and rebuild strength can be greatly impacted by making adequate and sensible food decisions. Proteins, vitamins, minerals, and other vital nutrients included in a well-balanced diet aid in tissue healing and help avert issues. Maintaining normal bladder function and reducing the risk of urinary tract infections require proper drinking.

Dietary adjustments may be necessary for post-operative nutrition, taking into account things like possible dietary limitations or changes in appetite. Preventing gastrointestinal discomfort can be achieved by including foods that are mild on the digestive system and easy to digest. Patients are frequently told to stay away from foods and drinks that could irritate their bladders or impede their ability to heal. Sustaining a wholesome and balanced diet throughout the recuperation phase might facilitate a more seamless healing procedure and enhance general health.

 Comprehending the healing process from bladder surgery entails being aware of the subtleties related to different surgical approaches and realizing the obstacles patients could encounter. Adherence to post-operative instructions, careful monitoring for complications, and an emphasis on diet to assist the body's healing mechanisms are all components of effective recovery management. The overall outcome of the bladder surgery journey can be improved by patients working together with healthcare experts during the post-surgical phase and by committing to a holistic approach to recovery.

CHAPTER TWO

GETTING READY FOR THE RECOVERING PROCESS

PRE-OPERATIVE NUTRITIONAL GUIDELINES

The Pre-Surgery Dietary Guidelines are essential for establishing the groundwork for a prosperous recuperation process. The decisions one makes about diet before surgery can have a big impact on how well the body heals and rebuilds strength.

It is best to concentrate on eating a range of nutrient-dense foods, such as fruits, vegetables, lean proteins, and whole grains, as part of a well-balanced diet. Consuming enough protein is especially crucial since it aids in tissue healing and aids in the body's reconstruction following surgery.

Including foods high in vitamins and minerals, such as zinc and vitamin C, can also help build a stronger immune system, which is crucial for healing after surgery.

THE VALUE OF HYDRATION

It is impossible to exaggerate the significance of staying hydrated when getting ready for the healing process. Maintaining proper hydration is essential for many physiological processes, such as the movement of nutrients, the removal of waste, and the upkeep of general body functioning. Drinking enough water can help avoid problems like constipation and improve circulation, both of which are essential for recovery. Water should be consumed regularly both before and after the operation, as advised by medical professionals. However, particular recommendations may change according to a patient's health history and the type of surgery, so speaking with medical professionals is crucial to adjusting hydration requirements.

MENTAL READINESS FOR RECUPERATION

A crucial part of the entire healing process, mental preparation for recovery is sometimes overlooked. It can help to mentally prepare for the obstacles that might come up during the healing process. Important aspects of mental preparation include recognizing the need for patience, identifying probable discomforts, and setting reasonable expectations.

Practicing mindfulness, meditation, or relaxation techniques can assist in reducing tension and anxiety related to the impending surgery and the healing time that follows. Creating a network of support that consists of loved ones, friends, and medical experts can help WITH emotional support and foster a more optimistic outlook, which will increase the resilience required to effectively complete the recovery process.

A comprehensive strategy for getting ready for the healing process includes not just physical but also nutritional and psychological elements. The Pre-Surgery Dietary Guidelines establish the foundation for ideal nutrition, guaranteeing that the body is prepared for effective healing. It is impossible to overstate the significance of being hydrated since healthy fluid balance is essential for several body processes that are vital to healing. Last but not least, Mental Preparation for Recovery is essential for developing resilience, controlling stress, and cultivating an optimistic outlook—all of which help the healing process go more smoothly and successfully.

CHAPTER THREE

ESSENTIAL POST-SURGERY DIETARY ITEMS

FIRST DIETARY GUIDELINES

Following the right dietary recommendations is essential for a speedy recovery following surgery. The first set of food instructions following surgery is crucial for accelerating recovery and averting problems. Focusing on foods that are high in nutrients and readily digested is crucial during the early phases as they supply the building blocks required for tissue regeneration and general recovery.

FOODS THAT ARE SOFT AND EASILY DIGESTED

To reduce the early post-surgery period's impact on the digestive system, soft, readily digestible foods are advised. These foods are easier for the body to digest, absorb, and use, and they are kinder to the stomach. Soups, broths, pureed veggies, yogurt, and cooked grains are a few examples of these meals. These choices not only facilitate easier digestion but also aid in avoiding any discomfort or problems that can result from consuming meals that are more difficult to digest.

It is crucial to include a range of foods high in nutrients in the post-surgery diet. Foods high in nutrients give the body the vital vitamins, minerals, and other elements it needs to assist its healing processes. A well-rounded and nourishing post-surgery nutrition plan should contain fruits and vegetables, whole grains, lean meats, and healthy fats. These meals support energy production, tissue repair, and immunological function—all vital components of the healing process.

WHY NUTRIENT-RICH FOODS ARE IMPORTANT

In the aftermath of surgery, the significance of staying hydrated cannot be emphasized enough. Drinking enough water is essential for several body processes, such as digestion, circulation, and waste product removal. Consuming enough fluids also lessens the risk of issues like constipation, which can often occur after surgery. To stay well hydrated, clear broths, herbal teas, and water are great options.

Furthermore, depending on the specific surgical procedure and the patient's health, dietary modifications can be required. People who have had gastrointestinal surgery or who have particular dietary limitations, for example, might need to adhere to customized rules.

To create a customized post-surgery food plan, close collaboration with medical specialists like nutritionists or dietitians is essential. Based on the patient's medical background, dietary habits, and unique recuperation requirements, these specialists can offer insightful advice. Maintaining regular contact with the medical staff increases the likelihood of a speedy and effective recovery by ensuring that the food plan is modified as necessary during the healing process.

CHAPTER FOUR

THE DIET PLAN SUITABLE FOR BLADDERS

MAKING A WELL-COMPOSED MEAL PLAN

For those who follow a bladder-friendly diet, developing a balanced meal plan is essential to controlling and reducing symptoms related to bladder disorders. The main objective is to include meals that are easy on the bladder while maintaining a healthy and balanced diet. To achieve this, a balance must be maintained between the various food groups, such as proteins, carbs, fats, and micronutrients.

A diet plan that is healthy for the bladder must emphasize lean proteins like fish, chicken, tofu, and lentils. These protein sources support the general health of muscles and are less likely to cause bladder irritation. Moreover, adding complex carbs from fruits, vegetables, and whole grains delivers necessary nutrients without irritating the bladder.

Add healthy fats for satiety and general well-being, such as those found in almonds, avocados, and olive oil.

FOODS TO TAKE AND LEAVE OUT

A range of vibrant fruits and vegetables should be included in the diet to improve its nutritional composition. These offer vital vitamins, minerals, and antioxidants that promote the general well-being of the body. Citrus fruits and tomatoes are examples of acidic fruits and vegetables that should be limited or avoided because they can aggravate bladder discomfort in certain people.

In addition, maintaining adequate fluids is essential for bladder health. While drinking enough water is important, it's a good idea to keep an eye on and modify your intake of potentially irritating liquids like tea, coffee, and acidic fruit juices. Drinking herbal teas or water flavored with mint or cucumber can be cooling substitutes for people trying to keep their bladders healthy.

It is equally vital to be aware of specific foods and beverages that may irritate the bladder while thinking about a bladder-friendly diet. These could include foods high in acidity, carbonated beverages, artificial sweeteners, and spicy foods. Individuals can better understand their triggers and adjust their meal plans by keeping a food diary.

EXAMPLE MENUS FOR VARIOUS REHAB PHASES

Individual tastes and dietary requirements can be taken into account when creating sample meal plans for various stages of rehabilitation. Simple and easily digested foods like grilled chicken, steamed veggies and plain rice may be included during the early phases of rehabilitation. More diversity, including a greater range of fruits, vegetables, and lean meats, can be included as patients grow better.

Later on, a well-rounded meal plan can include a variety of nutrient-dense foods with a focus on a balanced combination of proteins, carbs, and fats.

A handful of nuts, whole-grain crackers with hummus, or yogurt with low-acid fruits can all be considered snacks. The secret is to adjust the meal plans according to individual tolerance levels and reintroduce foods gradually to assess the influence of each food on bladder health.

A diet that is friendly to the bladder should carefully evaluate food selection to reduce irritation and promote general well-being. It's critical to develop a well-balanced diet plan that stays away from potential triggers and includes lean proteins, complex carbohydrates, and healthy fats. Meal plans that are customized for various phases of recuperation also guarantee a gradual return of meals, which aids in bladder health management.

CHAPTER FIVE

CONTROLLING TYPICAL POST-SURGERY SYMPTOMS WITH DIET

FEELING QUEASY AND THROWING UP

Common post-surgery symptoms that can have a serious impact on a patient's quality of life are nausea and vomiting. Numerous things, such as the use of anesthesia, painkillers, or the body's reaction to the surgical operation itself, could be the cause of these symptoms. The key to controlling nausea and vomiting with food is to eat gradually. Starting with simple, easily digested foods like crackers, plain rice, or broths is a common recommendation given to patients. Small, regular meals spread out throughout the day might lessen the chance of nausea and assist avoid overloading the digestive system.

It's critical for those who are suffering from nausea and vomiting to drink enough water in addition to making the correct dietary choices. Drinking clear liquids can help you stay hydrated. Examples of these are water, ginger tea, and electrolyte drinks. Eating lighter, properly cooked meals instead of large, oily ones will help the healing process go more smoothly. Additionally, patients should speak with their medical professionals about anti-nausea drugs that they can add to their post-surgery routine.

CONSTIPATION

Another typical post-surgery symptom that can be uncomfortable and interfere with healing is constipation. The use of painkillers, altered eating habits, and decreased physical activity are all major causes of post-operative constipation. Patients are advised to progressively increase their consumption of fiber to solve this issue through diet. Whole grains, fruits, vegetables, legumes, and other high-fiber foods can all aid in promoting regular bowel motions.

Both preventing and treating constipation depend on enough hydration. Getting enough water in your diet helps make feces softer and easier to move through the digestive system. It can also be helpful to include foods like prune juice or prunes that have inherent laxative qualities. However, before making big dietary adjustments after surgery, people should be aware of their unique dietary requirements and speak with medical experts.

HANDLING SHIFTS IN APPETITE

Handling changes in hunger is a complex component of healing after surgery that needs to be carefully considered. An individual's appetite may be affected after surgery for a variety of reasons, including changes in the digestive tract, pharmaceutical side effects, or stress. When this happens, it's critical to concentrate on eating a diet high in nutrients, which supplies vital vitamins and minerals to aid in the healing process.

To maintain a consistent food intake, patients who are experiencing changes in appetite may find it beneficial to eat smaller, more frequent meals throughout the day. Consuming meals high in protein, such as dairy, eggs, and lean meats, can help promote tissue healing and repair. Speak with a qualified dietitian or other healthcare professional for individualized advice on how to modify your diet throughout the post-surgery phase to suit your unique nutritional requirements.

A careful and customized strategy is needed to manage typical post-surgery symptoms through food. By choosing simple, easily digested foods and drinking plenty of water, nausea and vomiting can be prevented. Increases in fiber consumption over time, together with increased hydration and the use of natural laxatives, can help relieve constipation. It's important to prioritize nutrient-dense foods and frequent, smaller meals while managing fluctuations in appetite. All things considered, a customized and well-balanced diet after surgery is essential for facilitating a quicker recovery and maximizing the healing process.

CHAPTER SIX

FLUID INTAKE AND HYDRATION

THE SIGNIFICANCE OF HYDRATION FOR RECOVERY

Whether recovering from an illness, physical exercise, or other pressures on the body, hydration is essential. Consuming enough fluids is crucial to regaining and sustaining healthy body functions. The body loses more fluids during recuperation because of things like breathing, sweating, and higher metabolic activity.

The restoration of electrolyte balance, which is essential for muscular function, neuron communication, and general physiological well-being, depends on replacing these lost fluids.

It is especially clear how crucial hydration is to recuperation after physical activity. Exercises that are intense cause a person to perspire more, which causes them to lose electrolytes and water. Maintaining adequate hydration not only helps avoid dehydration but also lessens weariness and pain in the muscles. Drinking electrolyte-rich fluids during post-exercise recovery will help to replace lost sodium, potassium, and other vital minerals more quickly, which can speed up recovery and lessen the chance of cramps and spasms.

SELECTING THE PROPER DRINKS

One of the most important parts of being properly hydrated is selecting the right drinks. The most obvious and essential option is water, which is also an essential part of being hydrated. Its advantages go beyond simple hydration because water is necessary for proper digestion, nutritional absorption, and temperature regulation. Sports drinks, which also contain water, might be helpful while engaging in vigorous physical activity since they offer an additional source of carbohydrates and electrolytes. However, it is vital to be cautious of the sugar content in such beverages and choose ones that fit with specific hydration demands.

KEEPING AN EYE ON FLUID INTAKE

Since individual needs might vary depending on factors including age, weight, activity level, and climate, monitoring fluid intake is essential to maintaining hydration. Although thirst is a good indicator of when the body needs to refill its fluid supply, you shouldn't depend just on it. Making it a practice to check the color of your pee can provide important information about your level of hydration; lighter colors indicate you're well hydrated, while darker colors indicate you need to drink more fluids.

Healthcare practitioners may suggest particular hydration regimens for various conditions, such as illness or recuperation from specific medical operations. In severe circumstances, intravenous (IV) hydration may be used to guarantee quick fluid replacement. In these situations, it's critical to heed medical advice and instructions to customize fluid intake to meet individual demands.

Maintaining general health and well-being requires understanding the significance of hydration in recovery, choosing wisely when selecting beverages, and closely monitoring fluid intake. Maintaining proper hydration is essential for optimum physiological function and effective recuperation, regardless of the situation—physical activity, illness, or daily living.

CHAPTER SEVEN

SUPPLEMENTAL NUTRITION FOR IMPROVED RECUPERATION

SYNOPSIS OF SUPPLEMENTS

The provision of vital nutrients by nutritional supplements facilitates the body's healing processes, which is a critical factor in improving recovery. Knowing the various kinds of supplements and their advantages might help you develop a more successful recovery plan.

A person's diet can be supplemented with a variety of goods, such as vitamins, minerals, amino acids, and herbal extracts, which are intended to meet particular health needs.

These supplements are frequently used to fill up nutritional shortages, particularly when there is a rise in physical stress, illness, or injury recovery.

MINERALS AND VITAMINS FOR HEALING

Minerals and vitamins are essential for the body to cure itself. They serve crucial roles in tissue repair, immunological response, and general cellular health as well as serving as cofactors for a variety of enzymatic activities.

For example, vitamin C is well-known for its antioxidant qualities, which aid in the manufacture of collagen, which is essential for wound healing, and fight oxidative stress.

Minerals like magnesium and zinc are also essential to the recuperation procedure. Magnesium is important for energy production and muscular function, while zinc is essential in immune system function and protein synthesis. Increasing the amount of vitamins and minerals in one's diet or taking supplements might help improve the healing process considerably.

TALKING WITH MEDICAL PROFESSIONALS

But it's important to proceed cautiously with supplementation and consult medical professionals for advice. Speaking with a medical expert guarantees that the supplements selected are suitable for a person's unique requirements and do not adversely affect any prescription drugs or pre-existing medical issues. By providing tailored guidance based on a patient's medical history, healthcare professionals can guarantee the safe and efficient use of dietary supplements.

Take into account the person's general nutritional state and eating habits before adding any supplements to a rehabilitation plan. The cornerstone should always be a varied and well-balanced diet; supplements should be used to enhance a healthy lifestyle, not to replace it.

By supplying vital nutrients that aid in the body's mending processes, dietary supplements can significantly improve recuperation. Particularly, vitamins and minerals support several physiological processes that are essential for healing. To guarantee safety and efficacy, it is crucial to approach supplements cautiously and consult healthcare professionals. Optimizing the benefits of nutritional supplements for improved recovery requires a comprehensive strategy that includes speaking with medical specialists and putting an emphasis on a well-balanced diet.

CHAPTER EIGHT

PHYSICAL ACTIVITY AND EXERCISE DURING THE HEALING PROCESS

THE VALUE OF MODERATE EXERCISE

Recovering from disease or injury frequently necessitates striking a careful balance between rest and exercise. It is acknowledged that little exercise is an essential part of the recuperation process for several reasons. First of all, mild exercise encourages blood circulation, which helps the body's tissues receive vital nutrients and oxygen, speeding up the healing process. It also aids in preventing joint stiffness and muscular atrophy, two conditions that are frequently brought on by extended periods of inactivity.

The benefits of light exercise for mental health emphasize how important it is. The body's natural mood enhancers, endorphins, are released when you exercise. These endorphins can help you feel happier and reduce anxiety or depression symptoms that may come with your healing process. Additionally, light exercise encourages a proactive attitude to recovery by empowering oneself and providing a sense of accomplishment.

ADAPTED GUIDELINES FOR PHYSICAL ACTIVITY

The Modified Physical Activity Guidelines are essential for ensuring that people in the recovery stage exercise in a way that is suitable for their particular condition. These recommendations consider the person's general health, the type of disease or damage, and the degree of recuperation. Following the updated recommendations promotes a safe and efficient return to regular physical activity by lowering the chance of setbacks or aggravating pre-existing medical conditions.

INCLUDING EXERCISE IN EVERYDAY ROUTINE

Including exercise in everyday activities is crucial for encouraging a steady and progressive recovery. This method places a strong emphasis on incorporating low-intensity exercises, stretching, and walking into regular tasks. Through the integration of these activities into everyday routines, people can sustain a steady state of physical activity without going overboard. This not only helps the healing process but also encourages the formation of enduring habits that advance general well-being.

Additionally, including movement in everyday activities promotes a holistic approach to health. It is consistent with the idea that physical activity may be incorporated into many facets of daily life and is not just for scheduled workouts. This method not only helps patients recover but also lays the groundwork for a post-rehabilitation lifestyle that is more active and health-conscious.

It is impossible to exaggerate the value of mild activity during recovery. It is a versatile instrument that encourages mental health, physical recovery, and a proactive outlook. The Modified Physical Activity Guidelines provide a customized exercise program that is in keeping with each person's health status. Finally, integrating movement into everyday activities promotes a sustainable and all-encompassing approach to recovery and long-term well-being by extending the advantages of exercise beyond set workout sessions.

CHAPTER NINE

EMOTIONAL HEALTH IN THE PROCESS OF HEALING

HANDLING EMOTIONAL DIFFICULTIES

Whether recovering from physical illnesses, mental health problems, or addiction, emotional well-being is essential. It entails developing resilience, being aware of and in control of one's emotions, and cultivating an optimistic outlook that promotes recovery. Overcoming emotional obstacles in the course of recovery requires a comprehensive strategy that takes into account all aspects of a person's life.

Psychotherapy and counseling are examples of therapeutic procedures that can offer a secure environment for people to examine and express their feelings. These sessions aid in identifying the root causes of emotional discomfort and support the development of more healthy coping strategies in the participants.

Furthermore, combining mindfulness and relaxation methods can provide people with the ability to control and navigate their emotional reactions.

INTERACTION BETWEEN MOOD AND DIET

During recovery, emotional health is greatly influenced by the complex and dynamic interaction that exists between mood and diet. Foods high in nutrients are essential for maintaining neurotransmitter production and brain function, which in turn impacts mood and mental health in general. A healthy, well-balanced diet can help to stabilize mood, energy levels, and cognitive abilities.

Some nutrients, like zinc and magnesium, vitamins B and D, and omega-3 fatty acids, have been linked to reduced symptoms of anxiety and depression and increased mood. On the other hand, a diet heavy in sugar, processed foods, and bad fats might worsen mental health by causing inflammation. Thus, to support emotional resilience and overall well-being, people in recovery are urged to follow a diet rich in nutrients.

COPING MECHANISMS AND SUPPORT NETWORKS

Developing strong support networks and coping mechanisms is essential to overcoming emotional obstacles during the healing process. Emotional resilience can be increased by establishing healthy coping strategies like mindfulness training, physical activity, and creative expression.

These techniques provide people the ability to control their emotions, handle stress, and go through the highs and lows of the healing process.

Friends, family, and neighborhood organizations are examples of support networks that are essential to emotional health. Creating a network of sympathetic and understanding people gives one a sense of support and community. A collaborative approach to emotional rehabilitation can be fostered by peer support groups, therapy, and educational initiatives, which can provide insightful information and helpful coping mechanisms.

Managing emotional difficulties during the healing process necessitates a diverse strategy that includes therapy interventions, dietary concerns, and the development of coping mechanisms and support networks. Understanding how different facets of life are related to emotional health is crucial to promoting a comprehensive and long-lasting healing process.

CHAPTER TEN

LONG-TERM NUTRITIONAL ISSUES

MAKING THE SWITCH TO A REGULAR DIET

One of the most important aspects of long-term dietary considerations is making the switch to a regular diet, particularly for those who have had specific dietary treatments or have experienced health issues requiring temporary alterations. To establish durable habits and avoid any potential setbacks, the transition process should be executed with caution and graduality. This entails reintroducing a greater range of meals while being mindful of nutritional balance and quantity sizes. A licensed dietitian or healthcare professional consultation can offer tailored advice based on dietary preferences, personal health goals.

SUSTAINING A HEALTHFUL WAY OF LIFE

Long-term nutritional considerations go hand in hand with maintaining a healthy lifestyle. It includes more than simply the foods you choose; it also includes things like getting enough sleep, being hydrated, and engaging in regular physical activity. Taking a holistic approach to health can make a big difference in one's general well-being. It is possible to help meet nutritional needs by incorporating a wide variety of nutrient-rich foods, such as fruits, vegetables, whole grains, lean meats, and healthy fats. Exercise additionally helps to maintain weight control, improves mood, strengthens the heart, and increases vigor in general.

KEEPING AN EYE OUT AND PREVENTING RECURRENCE

Long-term dietary considerations must include both monitoring and preventing recurrence, especially for those who have had specific dietary interventions or have suffered health issues. Frequent medical examinations, which may include blood tests and other pertinent evaluations, can offer important insights into a person's general state of health. It's critical to continue to be on the lookout for any indications of recurrence and to take immediate action to address any new health issues. Furthermore, keeping lines of contact open with medical experts guarantees continued support and, if necessary, dietary plan modifications.

Long-term maintenance of favorable improvements in diet and health depends critically on understanding this relationship. A conscious and balanced diet combined with a dedication to an active lifestyle can make a big difference in one's general health and well-being. It's critical to see diet as a lifelong journey where individualized considerations, flexibility, and moderation are crucial to reaching and sustaining optimal health. In the end, the objective is to adopt a sustainable lifestyle that encourages longevity and vitality rather than merely making a brief adjustment.